Holistic Healing

Holistic Approach to Heal Yourself Naturally

Written by
Erik Penders

Amazon Kindle Edition

HOLISTIC HEALING

Copyright © 2015 by Erik Penders

TABLE OF CONTENTS

Book Description

This book has been created to give you a crash course in holistic remedies. I will explain the different sides of holistic remedies and what you can do to generally improve your health, reduce stress and many other benefits.

My passion is health, nutrition and the human body and mind. I love finding out how our bodies and our minds work. I do a lot of research in these areas. This book is one of many projects, where I share practical, researched information about a subject, in this case: "holistic remedies". I focus on giving you the most important information, I found in my research. So you instantly know you have the best information about this subject. Holistic remedies and holistic healing, in my opinion, is highly undervalued and in my experience many illnesses, injuries and ailments can be either prevented and/or cured by holistic healing and remedies. Because this is one of many subjects I write about, I want to let you know I don't just write about the subject. I don't "just" try to inform you with the best information. I also aim for practical, solution based information, that you can use straight away. You can find many practical, easy to follow tips, tricks and advice in this book to heal yourself with an holistic approach.

Happy reading and let me know your thoughts!

About the Writer

Hi, I'm Erik. Thank you so much for reading my work. I'm a fitness enthusiast and entrepreneur from the Netherlands. I've started working in this fitness industry at the age of 21. I've always had a big fascination about the human body and the way it works. Especially in combination with exercising and nutrition. I've started as a personal trainer and started my first business. I did quite well fortunately. After that I've started a bootcamp business in the city I live in (the hague) and it has grown to be the biggest in the Netherlands. Another one of my passions is sharing knowledge with others and as you can imagine I love to write about health topics, concerning the human body and nutrition. Although I'm probably not the best writer in the world (actually, I'm sure of that ;-)) I do however really aim for adding value to your life. If you can learn a few things from this book, I'm happy.

I know in this busy day and age, doing research takes to much of your time. So I love doing the work for you and share everything I've learned over the years and am still learning today. That's why you will not find any books from me about topics I'm not passionate about.

I hope you enjoy this book and it adds value to your life. If you find it interesting, feel free to share it with friends or family. You can also check out my other books and visit my website at: http://www.erikpenders.com

If you would be so kind to leave a review for this book, it will help me a lot in sharing this content.
It's totally fine to be honest, I'm confident that the information I share will add value to your life in one way or another.

Again, happy reading and I'd love to hear back from you on my website or in a review.

Erik.

Introduction

Holistic healing/holistic remedies basically means looking for alternative ways to heal yourself. Preferably natural, homeopathic ways. This kinda makes my happy, although not all medical and/or drug companies are necessarily wrong or evil, it's good to do your research. Without going to deep into what holistic healing is (you can find that in chapter 1) it focuses on the total body instead of a single part of it, with the physical, mental and emotional aspect combined. All holistic remedies you will find in this book are based on that principle.

We've all seen our body's capacity to heal itself in one way or another. This capacity is highly underrated and instead of fully utilizing this power many of us grab medicines and/or visit a doctor. In my experience, a lot of problems we encounter can either be prevented or cured by holistic remedies or at least being aware of your own power to heal yourself. Not only in general holistic remedies but also in holistic nutrition.

Good to know: For specific problems you should consult a (holistic) doctor. There is no problem in trying to heal yourself, but please be careful with specific problems. A professional is always recommended when facing issues you cannot resolve on your own.

Nature can do a lot for you, but I believe the emphasis in any holistic approach is on prevention, not necessarily treating and/or curing. You will find ways to treat yourself in this book, but I hope I've made my point.

What are Holistic Remedies

Holistic remedies are a certain way to heal, cure and/or treat injuries, ailments or illnesses. It sees al parts of the body as being interdependent to another. Even more so, it sees the body, mind, spirit and emotions as a whole. If one factor is out of balance, it affects the rest.

In my opinion it's not only about treatment it's even more about prevention. Living life "holistic" means you live in balance, all factors combined. The way to achieve this "balance" is easier said than done, I realize that. But there are a lot of ways to get there, and you'll find the most effective and important ones in this book. Don't forget that "balance" is relative. "Holistic" is relative as well.

This is what I mean: what we perceive generally healthy can differ from person to person. Although many similarities, there are also different perceptions about when you're truly living healthy or holistic. In my opinion you should focus on improvement, not being to drastic or to hard on yourself. Try to improve and enjoy the process is a different approach that can truly serve you. So, how do you know you're on the right track and how do you know you're improving in this area? It's actually quite simple. I'll tell you all about it, in the coming chapters.

Types of Holistic Remedies

Holistic remedy is a "broad concept". Which basically means there are a lot of different types of holistic remedies. First let me lay out the most important areas within holistic remedies.

- Holistic exercising
- Holistic nutrition
- Holistic medicine
- Holistic therapies

Let me give you some more details about these areas. Maybe unnecessary to mention that the four areas are not separate from each other. They are bound together. Most things I will mention under one of the four, will also (partly) apply for the other 3. Not all, but most. I will mention under the term what best suits the details and explanation about the mentioned info. Ok, enough about that. Let's dive in these four areas.

Holistic Exercising

One of the most obvious but also important parts in holistic remedies is exercising. There are a few types of exercising you can do. This is what holistic exercising can do for you in terms of benefits:

Increase you flexibility

- Relieve joint and muscle pain
- Strengthen and tone your body
- Balance your emotions
- Improve your sleep
- Enhance your circulation
- Improve digestion and bowel movement
- Calm your mind
- Boost your energy
- Regulate breathing
- Maintain general health
- Prevent ailments

Enough reason to start today I'm guessing. Now let me give you the possibilities in holistic exercising and show you how to use them. I'll also explain which type of exercising best suits particular goals. Here we go!

Yoga

This is by far the most important one in the area of exercising. Why? Yoga is one of the most balanced exercise styles you can find.

Although this is meant to be positive, some people experience this as a negative part of yoga. Yoga can sometimes seem a little bit "floaty" and too spiritual. Now of course there are still a lot of yoga practices that don't really feel right to grounded and objective people. But trust me, yoga is a great way to get a good workout and keep your body and mind balanced, which is crucial in holistic healing. Also more and more practices are getting less "floaty" and are getting increasingly enjoyable for grounded less spiritual people. Try it, until you find a practice that suits your personality and needs.

There are a lot of different types of yoga, here are the most practiced types with their most important features. Also I'll tell you which types of yoga are the most holistic. I believe it's best to find a practice with professionals, but you can do yoga at home as well. I'll give you some great resources to practice yoga at home. Here we go:

Kundalini Yoga: This is the most holistic type of yoga. Certain breathing techniques are used to clear your system and let energy flow through your body. Focused on chakra's and energy centers in the body, kundalini yoga is not necessarily about a workout, but more about energy.

Silvananda Yoga: Second most holistic is silvananda. Great for beginners because of the variety and many different parts of this style. Breathing exercises, relaxation, meditation, and different poses, everything is addressed in this style.

Hatha Yoga: A pretty "basic" type of yoga and the most common type. It mostly contains basic postures and the intensity is not really high.

Vinyasa Yoga: Fluid movements and smooth transitions from pose to pose describes this type of yoga. Vinyasa usually has a high intensity and lacks a "steady routine", instead you never know what's coming in Vinyasa yoga.

Ashtanga Yoga: One of the ancient styles of yoga. Ashtanga is similar to Vinyasa but has a specific sequence of poses. Ashtanga is a physically demanding style where the exact same poses in the same sequence are executed.

Iyengar Yoga: In this style of yoga "alignment" is the key factor. It's all about getting into a pose and holding that pose for a longer time, with emphasis of having proper alignments in the whole body.

Bikram Yoga: Gained in popularity over the last years, this style of yoga is done in a heated room. You follow the same sequence of poses and sweat a lot, really a lot. This style is loved by a big audience and seem to have reached the "mainstream" more than any other style of yoga.

Hot Yoga: A well known style of yoga. It's quite similar to Bikram, the sequences differ a little bit but the basis is the same. You will sweat ALOT.

As i mentioned before, I recommend you doing yoga with professionals. They will help you with the postures and the right execution of the yoga style you choose. You can find yoga classes everywhere. They are being offered worldwide and I bet there is a practice not very far from your house. Well maybe it's harder when you live in the countryside. Everybody's different so I cannot advise any of these types, since I don't know you. They're all equally good, depending on your wants and need. For this it's also best to try and find out for yourself based on the information I provided.

Yoga at Home

To do yoga on your own at your home, or basically anywhere, is definitely possible. I recommend visiting a few websites to find out more about doing yoga at home. It's actually important to keep some youtube films or pictures available during your yoga workout. So you can check if you're doing it right.

Here are some good resources I found for home yoga. Visit these websites:

http://www.wikihow.com/Do-Yoga-at-Home

https://yogainternational.com/article/view/the-beginners-guide-to-home-yoga-practice

A nice youtube video for yoga beginners is this one: https://www.youtube.com/watch?v=v7AYKMP6rOE

Hoping this links keep working, you never know when they take something offline. I think you get the idea, it's actually quite simple to find some good resources to do yoga at home.

Tai Chi

This is another great option. Tai chi is a form of martial arts. Although in most cases the exercise component is found more important. Which is understandable, but if you learn tai chi you will also learn very good self defense techniques.

Sometimes tai chi is described as "meditation in motion". It involves a series of movements, performed in a slow focused manner.

I won't go to far in depth with tai chi, preference is trying this form of exercising and see if it suits you and if you like it. Tai chi has 5 different styles, they all have their own methods and principles.

- Chen style

- Yang style
- Wu style
- Wu hao style
- Sun style

Again, getting into these different styles won't really serve you in my opinion. Trying tai chi in general will be the best way to determine if you like it and which style suits you the best.

Qigong and Traditional Chinese Exercising

Qi (pronounced "chee") means life force or vital energy that flows through all living things. Gong means accomplishment or skill through steady practice. Together (Chee gung) is generally explained as a system practiced for health maintenance, healing and increasing vitality.

It is often perceived in the west as a combination of martial arts and yoga. It shares an emphasis on gentle movements, flexibility and breathing. With many "yoga-like" movements and postures.

How to: Holistic Exercising

1. Choose to really dedicate yourself to try something new.
2. Realize that every new thing takes effort to start, block out any other possibility besides really trying this.
3. Choose on of the exercise forms that seems most appealing to you
4. Find a local practice or find a "home course" via google

5. Execute at least three lessons before deciding if it's for you

6. If you like it great, try to find a rhythm/habit to practice it regularly. If it's not for you, you still did an awesome job. You dedicated to trying and you did.

7. Repeat step 1 tot 6.

Holistic Nutrition

Holistic nutrition mostly focusses on "whole foods". It emphasizes a natural approach to nutrition and the body as a whole. Meaning that your nutrition influences not just one part of your body, but the whole body. Important in holistic nutrition is that your food is mostly in organic state. This means unrefined, unprocessed and preferably locally grown whole foods. If you decide to strive for holistic nutrition you will experience amazing benefits like:

- Improved skin
- Weight loss/weight management
- Improved mood
- Improved sleep
- Stronger immune system
- Balanced blood sugar levels
- Improved bowel and digestion
- Increased energy levels
- Reduced blood pressure

You should mostly focus on finding foods in their natural state. Deep in your gut you know that's what we're meant to eat. These are the products you should go for when you're aiming for a holistic diet:

- Vegetables (any kind!)
- Fruit, preferably combined with protein and healthy fats
- Nuts
- Seeds

- Chicken
- Turkey
- Eggs
- Oats
- Lean quark (if you're not lactose intolerant)
- Yoghurt (if you're not lactose intolerant)
- Oats
- Avocado's (mentioned separately because of the health benefits)
- Fish (omega 3, 6 and 9)

Also very important is to drink (filtered) water.

Tip! Please don't drink out of plastic bottles, since they do harm your health. Only bottles specially made for re-use should be used more than once. The plastic inside the bottles will release and end up inside your body.

Although this book is not about diet, I do want to give you some practical action steps to start with holistic nutrition today. (If you do want to go deeper into your diet, please visit my website and read more about nutrition and diet: http://www.erikpenders.com)

How to: Holistic Nutrition
1. Find recipes for the ingredients mentioned above.
2. Determine your day to day meals, which means meals you will eat more often than once. For instance: Breakfast: Oats, with

yoghurt, blueberries and honey. Write down at least 5 or 6 meals.

3. Make a grocery list and shop for these items.

4. Never shop for one meal, think "bulk" which means, any meal you prepare you prepare to eat 2 to 4 times from it. Leave leftovers in the fridge or freezer

5. Do not cut out all "bad habits" in your nutrition, that's unrealistic. Instead reward yourself for the work you've done. Automatically you will do this less and less.

6. Don't think to much about it, do this because you like taking care of yourself.

7. Keep telling yourself: "I'm doing this for me, for my health, my body and my life"

In my experience as a personal trainer, the best way to start with any type of diet or nutrition change, it all starts in between your ears. I don't care what people will tell you, it always takes commitment and effort and it's never easy. The best way to start is to really find out way you want to change. Make it so drastic, that you say to yourself: ENOUGH! This has to change NOW. Not a should, not a maybe, but a must. That's when you're willing to put in the effort and commit yourself to the change.

Next you need a plan, a plan that YOU need to make based on everything you learn. In this book, but also in the many many good resources you can find online and in other books.

Please remember than beginnings are always hard and take effort. The right time doesn't magically appear and it doesn't get easier tomorrow. All you need to focus on is forcing yourself towards the first step.

!Tip! In plenty of studies done on procrastination it's obvious that we should not focus on the task ahead, instead we should focus on the first, ridiculously small first step. If you want to stop after that first step, it's fine. Come back tomorrow and repeat. Trust me on this, it works! See what happens...

Holistic Medicines

In this section I want to tell you about the most impressive results with "alternative medicines" I have encountered in my research. Trying any of these if at your own risk and I do recommend you to look for a professional to use any of these medicines.

I personally believe in a lot of these medicines and I think they can be incredibly powerfull. From curing cancer, to losing weight, to healing skin to hundreds and hundreds more ailments or problems you have. Still, never lose your common sense and stay critical about everything. If you want to know more about any type of holistic medicine, look it up on the internet and again, be very wary for false information. There is a lot on the internet and you should research it well.

So here we go! There are a lot of health benefits for every single on mentioned below. But I'll just give a short description:

1. Weed oil or marijuana
Benefits: Too many to mention.

Perhaps you know it, perhaps you think I'm crazy. But I'm clearly not. I encounter hundreds, if not thousands of people really benefitting from weed oil. Keep in mind that in most countries it's illegal. Please consult your countries laws and rules before doing anything you might regret later.

I won't go into the details about this "wonder oil" but please feel free to research more if you want to. I cannot go into details, because there can be a whole separate book about it. I'm just letting you know, so you can find out more if you want to.

2. Aloe vera

Benefits: Aloe vera is also called a "wonderplant" because of it's healing properties. The gel inside the plants is generally used the treat cuts, burns and other skin conditions.

3. Ginger

Benefits: Known as one of the most powerful antioxidants ginger should be part of your daily diet. Ginger helps regulate blood flow and has many anti-inflammatory properties.

4. Garlic

Benefits: According to the american journal of clinical nutrition, garlic lowered rates of many different cancer forms. It also contains phytochemical which decrease high blood pressure.

5. Turmeric

Benefits: Contains Curcumin a powerful anti-inflammatory.

6. Cinnamon

Benefits: Anti-inflammatory, anti-cancer, blood sugar control, brain function and many many more

7. Globe artichoke

Benefits: Reduces cholesterol, heals your liver, reliefs irritable bowel syndrome and increases intestine and pancreatic health

8. Echinacea

Mostly used to treat and prevent catching a cold. But also increases interferon, fights cancer and fights infections in open wounds.

9. Sea buckthorn

Very healthy because of the high amount of vitamine C, but also protein, fibre, antioxidants and minerals. Totally jam-packed with healthy bioactive compounds.

10. Peppermint

Helps with a lot of different issues in the body, but one of the most prominent are digestion and bowel problems. From IBS, to cancer, to colonic spams, gastric disorders, you name it.

11. Ginseng

Anti-aging, mental stimulant, erectile disfunction's, blood sugar levels and much more.

12. Sage

Improves memory, prevents alzheimer, is anti-inflammatory and helps relieve diabetes type 2.

How to Use Holistic Medicines

To use any of these "alternative medicines", this is what you do:

1. First do more research about the holistic medicine you want to use. Either consult a professional or do the research on your own. Before you're absolutely sure about how to use it, don't. Of course in the list mentioned in this you can find plenty that will not require extensive research. But still, please be skeptical and consult a professional of you are not sure about whether to use it, or how to use it.

2. Depending on what you're using, always start with the smallest dose. This is not needed for natural herbs and plants without side effects. But of course I cannot predict what your needs are and what kind of medicine you will use and what it will be for.

3. When unsure, consult a professional. I cannot emphasize that enough. Especially with holistic medicines with severe side effects.

Holistic Therapies

Colon Therapy

Colon therapy is used to clean out the colon from undigested food that build up inside. It is believed to poison the body. Although there's not a lot of research done on this subject, many people claim that colon therapy works.

Before taking any drastic measures like going to a "colon therapist" I recommend you first try to clean your colon through nutrition.

How to: Colon Therapy

1. Double your water intake. Preferably drink mineral water and don't re-use plastic bottles.
2. Double your fiber intake. The more fiber you eat, the cleaner you colon will become. It's the only nutrient that is not digested and will support the bowel movements. Great resources are veggies, fruit, oats and seeds
3. Eat fermented foods. Bacterias in fermented foods suport digestion. Great resources are yoghurt and sauerkraut.
4. Focus on green vegetables. Chlorophyll is a substance that gives plants their green color, but also heals and soothes your digestive track.
5. More physical activity. Taking the stairs more often, going for a lunch walk or taking the bike instead of the car makes a big difference. Physical activity

6. Use (natural) supplements to clean your colon. Before taking up this option, please consult a doctor. You can find these supplements in any health and drugstore, but go informed. Not everything is safe, especially in combination with other drugs/medicines.

Metabolic Therapy

This therapy is made to cure imbalance caused by the buildup of toxic substances. It's quite similar to colon therapy, but it's goal is not necessarily to cure the colon, but to let the body be able to heal itself. The focus with this is therapy is also natural "whole" foods, that will detoxify your body. Metabolic is often referred to as "anti-cancer" therapy. It is believed, although not subject in a lot of research, that metabolic therapy cleanses the body from toxins and wastes. To do metabolic therapy on your own is hard and complex. Because of the drastic and sometimes vigorous measures, I truly recommend to consult a professional before trying this therapy. Metabolic therapy is most done through these main areas:

- Therapeutic nutrition
- Supplements
- Vigorous detoxification

Therapeutic nutrition and supplements is quite possible to do on your own. Vigorous detoxification is not. A few practical things done in vigorous detoxification are for instance coffee enema's and organ flushes.

How to: Metabolic Therapy

An other approach to metabolic therapy is for "low metabolic energy", which many people suffer from. Most common symptoms for low metabolic energy are:

- Feeling tired or worn down
- Trouble sleeping
- Troubles with weight management
- Feeling cold most of the times
- Dry skin
- Memory problems

The are a few reasons for low metabolic energy. The thyroid gland plays a part as it cannot make enough T4, which is hypothyroidism. Also the adrenal glands often have trouble handling the normal metabolic energy created by your body and force a down regulation. Hormonal imbalances also play a role and severe calorie restriction.

If you recognize any of the symptoms listed above, this is what you can do by yourself, before consulting a doctor and/or professional:

- Reduce stress

Stress is the biggest enemy of your adrenal glands. Stress is a broad subject, you might be suffering from it without knowing. The opposite of stress is helpful and will help you reduce stress. Think rest, joy, peace, sleep, relaxation, stability, peace.

• Improve nutrition

There it is again. Nutrition is vital in general, but specifically for this you need to:
  • Eat more protein
  • Reduce carbs (mostly sugars)
  • Reduce stimulants like caffeine, alcohol and cigarettes

Also these supplements will help you:
  • B-complex
  • Amino acids
  • Omega 3,6,9 (fish oil)
  • Unrefined sea salt

Perhaps you find a common factor in different parts in this book. I cannot emphasize enough how important "Good nutrition" is. Not only generally speaking, but also for very specific problems with and inside your body and even your mind. It affects everything. An holistic way of thinking is complementary to that thought and in my opinion, it's 100% true. Think about this: "How can it not influence everything, if you would only look at the miracle of how our bodies function".

!Tip! With being skeptical about what you put in your body, you're half way there. Read labels and see how many 'abracadabra' words are on the ingredient list. You'll be amazed how easy you can find better options.

Acupuncture

Although there are not many scientific studies about acupuncture, again many people experience benefits from it. Acupuncture comes from traditional chinese medicine. It involves inserting tiny needles into the body. This needles are places on acupuncture points or acupoints, which are often located close to meridians. These are connected points in your body that affect specific organs or parts of the body.

Acupuncture is most often used for the relief of any kind of pain. Although according to some people acupuncture is very effective it is mostly used to adjunct other forms of treatment.

It is still described as "pseudoscience" because of the lack of evidence that it truly works. Still, it's worth trying if you want to go over your options. Let me tell you how.

How to: Acupuncture

I can be quite brief about this section. You cannot do acupuncture on your own and you need to go to a clinic. I do however recommend you don't rush it and look for a good one. Preferably one where you find more than 10 customer reviews and check how long they've been working in this field. How long have they been practicing acupuncture and what is the background of the staff working there. Might sound as an open door, but it's still important to do this!

Reiki

Reiki is a Japanese technique based on "life energy" It claims that when your life energy is low you are more at risk to get sick or unable to fully enjoy life. It claims to reduce stress, enhance relaxation and that it assists healing. I've personally never tried Reiki, but with this method you can also find a lot of people claiming they benefit from it.

Reiki is made up of two Japanese words. Rei, which means "the higher power" and ki which means "life energy" So complete you can interpret is as: "A higher power guided life force energy"

For reiki also counts it treats the whole person, body, mind, spirit and emotions. People experiencing a Reiki treatment feel a glowing radiance and warmth through and over the entire body.

My opinion is that I'm open for any kind of "natural healing" and I think so should you. I haven't experienced it yet, but because it's a simple, safe and natural method of spiritual healing, it's safe to try it.

How to: Reiki

Same as acupuncture there is no real way to do Reiki on your own. So if you're open to try this, than find a professional practice that has a proven track record as being professional and enjoyable for their customers.

Aromatherapy

A french perfumer and chemist started with the term "aromatherapy" in 1937. it is often referred to as utilizing "essential oils" which is a different term but means about the same.

In aromatherapy you will experience a therapeutic application or medical use of aromatic substances, e.g essential oils. The last 20 years aromatherapy has become more and more holistic. So nowadays it also approaches the whole body, mind, spirit and emotions. Mostly used to support he body's natural ability to be balanced and stay balanced. Not necessarily treating one ailment or injury, rather letting the body heal itself by restoring balance. Without getting to much into aromatherapy, I can actually share with you how you do aromatherapy on your own, at home.

A great upside of this therapy is that anyone can use it, anywhere. You just need the right ingredients. So let me give you some very practical ways to experience and enjoy aromatherapy.

How to: Aromatherapy

I'm just going to give you practical information here. You can find the mentioned oils in most health stores, ordering on the internet is also a great option.

A few of the oils most commonly used:

- Lavender oil
- Sage oil
- Jojoba oil
- Lemon oil
- Rosemary oil
- Basil oil
- Bergamot oil
- Tea tree oil
- Eucalyptus oil
- Peppermint oil
- Jasmine oil
- Chamomile oil

You can use oil of this oils as you please, that's the beauty of the aromatherapy. It's perfectly fine to experiment a little bit and find what you like. Nevertheless, I will tell you what these herbs are mostly used for. Again, you don't have to stick to what's listed below, experiment to your liking!

Lavender oil

Good for: Relieve tension, burns, stings and your skin in general.
Mostly used for: fighting headaches, stress, hypertension, skin problems, massages.

Sage oil

Good for: Anti bacterial, soothing and relaxing.

Mostly used for: Skin conditions, decreasing stress.

Jojoba oil

Good for: Skin, cleansing, muscle care.

Mostly used for: Massages, skin care.

Lemon oil

Good for: Anti bacterial, anti viral and anti histamine.

Mostly used for: Infections, sore throats, nail care, skin care, small cuts.

Rosemary oil

Good for: Indigestion, Stress relief, pain relief.

Mostly used for: Constipation, bloating, muscle pain and even arthritis.

Basil oil

Good for: infections, blood sugar, stress reduction.

Mostly used for: As antibiotic for infections, stings and bites and colds.

Bergamot oil

Good for: Infections, skin cuts and wounds, muscle cramps.

Mostly used for: Calming nervous system, depression, skin and anti-inflammatory properties.

Tea tree oil

Good for: bacterial and viral infections, cuts and wounds.

Mostly used for: Sort throats, ear aches, skin care and insect repellent.

Eucalyptus oil

Good for: Concentration, detoxification, relieving pain.

Mostly used for: Colds, skin problems like itching and bug bites, infections.

Peppermint oil

Good for: Soothing, cooling, muscle care.

Mostly used for: Treating stomach issues, air deodorizer, concentration.

Jasmine oil

Good for: Revitalization, energie, anti depressant

Mostly used for: soothing and calming in general.

Chamomile oil

Good for: Skin conditions, inflammation

Mostly used for: Skin problems, sleeping problems, stomach problems.

Meditation

This part might be more important than you think. Why?

1. Many researchers claim it's potentially one of the most effective forms of stress reduction.
2. Stress reduction techniques in the western world are claimed to be less effective and at least not consistently effective.

Meditation techniques you will find do not emphasize the true nature and meaning of meditation. Meditation can be described as a state of thoughtless awareness. It's not just imagining something that gives us a feeling of peace or satisfaction. It's also not about stopping the mind all together. More so it's not about concentration, certain exercises or mental effort. To give you an idea: Someone can be in a state of meditation in a crowded room with a lot of noise, while someone can be far from meditation in a lotus posture on a quiet field in the forest. So before you want to try meditation, it's important to know what it really is. The best description of meditation according to me personally and which I found in researching the subject is this:

"Meditation is a state of thoughtless awareness, without effort, with a focus on the present moment"

Which techniques do I recommend and how do you practice meditation? Let me show you:

How to: Meditate

Although there are many different forms of meditation, science doesn't really show a difference in outcome or results. Also the experiences are very divided in what works for who. So it's all about finding out what works best for you if you want to try meditation. Let me help you to start!

I will not go into the different types of meditation, I'd rather just tell you how to do it. Of course if you want to find out, you can look it up on google. So here we go!

Please not that when trying meditation for the first time, you might experience discomfort or unease with sitting still and keep your attention inside yourself. But that will get better. A candle in front of you can help. Make sure the location is peaceful and quiet.

1. Find a place where you can sit quietly and comfortably, without being disturbed.
2. When you've settled down, take your attention slowly to the top of your head.
3. When experiencing a slight tingle in your hands and/or your spine you're on the right track. Don't worry about the thoughts still in your mind, let it be. Keep the focus on the top of your head.
4. After 10-15 minutes you're done.

Now this may seem a little bit weird and I'm sure you didn't experience a magical meditation the first time. Which is totally fine! Repeat this sequence daily and see what happens...

It's not about rushing it, it's also not about criticizing yourself. Take the time and just see it as a moment to relax.

Conclusion

I truly hope you have enjoyed reading this book. I've mentioned the best holistic remedies and ways of healing I found in my research. Most of the described techniques you can try on your own, since they are safe, natural and easy to use. Others I've mentioned and recommended to consult a professional. Which you should do, before trying any of those options.

I hope this book will add value to your life and if you've enjoyed the information I would very much appreciate you leaving an awesome review of the book. Thanks in advance, you're really helping me out with it.

Also, if you have any interest in more health related topics and/or writing from me, visit my website: http://www.erikpenders.com.

As I mentioned before I write about a lot of subjects related to health, the human body and nutrition. As I've told you in the section "about the writer" I've been a personal trainer in the past and my field of expertise is weight loss and body mechanics.

I want to thank you again, for downloading this book. It gives me a great feeling that I can reach anyone across the ocean, in major cities and small villages. What a blessing.

Take care, have an awesome day and cheers to you,

Erik